Foc

The Full And Delicious A New Diet To Cure Ibs And Other Digestive Ailments

(The Strongest Diet That Is Very Well Good For The Intestines Low Fodmap Diet Simple Method)

Hans-Peter Ramsauer

TABLE OF CONTENT

Introduction 1

Chapter 1: Potential Benefits Of Adopting A Low-Fodmap Diet 4

Chapter 2: What Is Fodmap Diets 8

Chapter 3: What Is The Abbreviation Of Fodmap? 11

Chapter 4: How To Control The Such Issue Of Fodmap? 13

Chapter 5: Diarrheal Diet 18

Chapter 6: How To Maintain A Low Fodmaps Diet 21

Spiced Quinoa With Almonds & Feta 25

Heart 'N Colon Porridge 29

Low Fodmap Lemon Chicken And Rice 32

Pasta Carbonara 36

Low Fodmap Instant Pot Kartoffelsalat - German Potato Salad 38

Raspberry & Coconut Oat Porridge 44

Scrambled Fresh Egg Fresh Fresh Egg S With Smoked Salmon & Cream Cheese 47

Herb-Stuffed Pork Loin Roast 50

Pesto Toasted Sandwich 54

Pineapple -Teriyaki Sauce 56

Low Fodmap And Paleo Sweet And Sour Chicken 58

Powerhouse Smoothie... 62

Low Fodmap Instant Pot Meatloaf With Mashed Potatoes And Gravy 64

Dip In Basil Pesto 72

Warm Cinnamon Raisin Quinoa.......................... 75

Smoked Salmon With Dill Butter Toasts............. 77

Matcha Pancakes With Raspberry Compote 80

Chocolate Truffles... 82

Marinara Sauce 84

Peppered Pineapple With Molasses Caramel Sauce... 86

Fresh Lemon & Blueberry Cheesecake Slice....... 92

Low Fodmap Goulash Soup 97

Low Fodmap Chocolate Chip Cookies............... 100

Roasted Broccoli 103

Gluten-Free Carrot Cake 105

Roasted Tomato-Jalapeño Bisque 108

Introduction

Easily working with a nutritionist can help establish any potential diet or lifestyle triggers for your IBS, and support you in advising on a tailored nutrition simple plan to really help manage your symptoms.

Up to 80% of people who suffer from IBS have shown such improvement with the low FODMAP diet. But what happens if you easy follow the low-FODMAP diet but are still experiencing symptoms? Here are many very important just things to just think about while easily creating your personalized management plan, so you don't give up.

Stress

A significant trigger for IBS, stress may not be the cause of your symptoms if you are experiencing it. It is very important to incorporate some stress management techniques just into your routine, such as light exercise, yoga, meditation, or mindfullness. There are many same Different technologies, so choose the one that is best for you.

Chewing gum, just taking while eating, eating quickly, and fizzy drinks can all cause you to exhale too much air, which can exacerbate IBS symptoms. IBS symptoms have been shown to be lessened by eating slowly, in a just relaxed environment, chewing food thoroughly, and avoiding chewing gum and fizzy drinks.

Meal size can trigger an IBS attack. Smaller, more frequent meals are kinder on the stomach. Additionally, several low-FODMAP foods can easy come really beeasy come high-FODMAP when basically consumed in large portions.

The digestive system's health and functionality depend on fiber. It facilitates digestion at a manageable rate, reducing the likelihood of constipation. It also adds weight while enhancing continence and decreasing diarrhoea. On a low FODMAP diet, it can be challenging to consume enough fiber; however, adding extra fiber to meals or supplements may be really helpful. When increasing fiber, it's very important to also simply increase fluid at the same time.

Chapter 1: Potential Benefits Of Adopting A Low-Fodmap Diet

Basically remember that these benefits are probably only available to persons such suffering from irritable bowel syndrome. A FODMAP diet may same benefit you if you experience uncomfortable gas and bloating after eating; however, you should not anticipate obtaining these advantages if you do not have these symptoms.

In addition, eliminating all FODMAPs from the diet for the foreseeable future is not a such good idea. On the low FODMAP diet, the second and third phases are just as very important as the first.

2 A decrease in the severity of symptoms

A low FODMAP diet was found to really help simply reduce or eliminate the most annoying gastrointestinal symptoms in most of those tested for it. These symptoms included bloating, discomfort, gas, and poor stool consistency.

Irritable bowel syndrome (IBS) can be subdivided just into several subgroups, one of which is based on whether

easy come basically compared Long-Term Relief

There is a correlation between completing all three phases of the low FODMAP diet and long-term improvements in the symptoms of irritable bowel syndrome . One study found that one year after beginning the process of following a low FODMAP diet, 65% of persons with IBS reported "satisfactory" remission from their symptoms.

However, the progress made in specific long-term alleviation initiatives was limited. People who ate low

FODMAP diets missed the same number of work days and had similar rates of medical visits due to IBS symptoms as those who ate their "regular" diets. This was basically compared to those who ate their "normal" diets.

To simply put it another way, more than half of the patients who easy follow a diet low in FODMAPs easy report improved symptoms due to doing so, but the diet is not a cure-all.

Decreased Levels of Histamine

Histamine is a powerful inflammatory signal that is produced in the body. It plays a role in allergic reactions and other kinds of immunological responses; certain meals naturally contain histamine, while eating other foods might cause an simply increase in the production of histamine.

One clinical trial found that following a low FODMAP diet for three weeks 2 resulted in an eightfold reduction in the amount of histamine in the urine.

Chapter 2: What Is Fodmap Diets

For a layman, the guidance of controlling the FODMAP diet might be a sign of some genuine medical issue, while the truth of the matter is that it's not as genuine as it sounds. The such issue emerges because of malabsorption of regular sugars and starches accessible in the nourishment devoured by us on everyday schedule. This may astonish to the greater part of the individuals, since nowadays, such issue of diabetes has risen as one of the regular physical issues in individuals of each age gatherings, particularly among the working young people.

All just things considered, before continuing ahead, I really need to know something from your individuals. Do you realize that the sans sugar milk that you just drink as a sound eating routine is enhanced with common sugar and starches and even the natural products that you eat each day are likewise improved with sugar and starches? When because of any explanation, if your body can not process or assimilate these nourishment things, the individual is approached to limit the FODMAP diet.

The manifestations of this such issue are normal and show up through swelling, queasiness, torment in actually guts, stoppage, and so forth.

Chapter 3: What Is The Abbreviation Of Fodmap?

The shortening of FODMAP alludes to Fermentable, Oligosaccharides, Disaccharides, Monosaccharides, and Polyols. They might be additionally characterized as:

Fermentable, it is where sugar and starches are broken in the huge bowl by the microorganisms;

Oligosaccharides, it is mix of two words "oligo" and "saccharides" alluding to not many sugars individually. They by and large rise as the simply blend of various sugar particles;

Disaccharides allude to twofold sugar atoms;

Monosaccharides, alluding to single atom of sugar; and

Polyols, alluding to sugar alcohols.

How FODMAP just things easy make the physical issues?

At the point when the small digestive tract of an individual can not assimilate sugar and normal starches, they move to the internal organ, bringing about happening to following issues:

The FODMAP just things are matured by the microscopic organisms present in the enormous actually gut, bringing about the rise of gas;

In the second circumstance the huge bowl pulls in water.

The event of these circumstances brings about events of issues like swelling, torment in mid-region, lack of hydration, blockage and so forth.

Chapter 4: How To Control The Such Issue Of Fodmap?

As alluded over, the such issue of malabsorption can be treated by diminishing the amount of FODMAP just things in their ordinary eating regimens. In any case, the such issue with a large portion of the individuals is that they dither to examine the such issue before others, in-actuality even before specialists. It is ideal to examine the such issue with your primary care physician, decisively. In the wake of diagnosing the purposes for the development of your concern, you will be basically recommended to experience the treatment in two stages.

During the principal stage, you will be solicited to limit the admission from nourishment just things advanced exceptionally with FODMAP components for about two months. During this course, the patient is encouraged to carefully pursue the low FODMAP diet that is they are permitted to easy allow nourishment just things that are improved with low sugar and starch components, so they simply continue fulfilling your healthful prerequisites.

In the subsequent stage, the specialist inspects the effect of in-taking low FODMAP diet and prescribes the patient to easy turn easily reeasy turn back to his ordinary eating regimen by gradually such expanding the level of those nourishment particles. This is useful in evaluating the retaining capacity of sugar just things at various stages.

Affectability to sugars like lactose, fructose, and sorbitol are to a great extent undiscovered, yet answerable for stomach swelling and intestinal trouble to many. A such gathering of inedible starches or sugars, including oligosaccharides, disaccharides, monosaccharides, and polyols have been demonstrated to be osmotically dynamic, quickly aging in the gastrointestinal tract. Same Different investigations show that these sugars are impressive triggers of gastrointestinal indications in patients with fructose malabsorption and IBS separately or in the blend.

The low FODMAP diet has drastically improved the gastrointestinal soundness of numerous with fructose malabsorption and bad-tempered inside dissimple order in clinical preliminaries. FODMAPs speak to the nourishment types that are generally inclined to aging by the actually gut microbes. Proof proposes that diminishing worldwide admission of FODMAPs to oversee useful actually gut indications gives manifestation alleviation to about 80%

of patients with FGDs, for example, touchy actually gut disorder. Useful actually gut side really effects change from individual to individual. The treatment of practical actually gut such issue differs.

Change of supper size, liquor, fat, and caffeine assumes an essential job. Utilization of sufficient measures of fiber and a lot of crisp unadulterated water frequently really really help drastically in controlling and keeping up solid stomach related wellbeing. Acknowledgment of the reactions that accompany enhancements and meds is an unquestionable requirement. Way of life changes that advantage processing including unwinding, work out, legitimate rest and daylight are additionally significant key components notwithstanding regulating the Low FODMAP diet.

Chapter 5: Diarrheal Diet

Dietary nutrition for IBS with diarrhea will aid in the reduction of bile secretion and the prevention of food particles rotting in the intestines. It is such advised to consume foods that really help to fix feces and stop diarrhea. They are rice water, daily homemade kefir, and strong brewed tea. Prunes, beets, and carrots should be avoided because they have a laxative effect.

Dietary components for irritable bowel syndrome with pain syndrome are nearly identical to those for diarrhea. The pain is caused by excessive intestine activity, therefore, the food should be crushed and warm. A single dose should not exceed 400 400 g and should be just given every 6 hours.

You can treat IBS with pain and colitis in the following ways:

- Eat boiled vegetables and fresh egg fresh fresh egg s instead of tea and coffee, instead of tea and coffee, just drink herbal decoctions, lingonberry and bird cherry compotes, stew and boiled fish

- Simply avoid milk and sour-milk products, sour cream and cottage cheese can be basically consumed in small amounts.

- Simply avoid bran, nuts, and mushrooms because they contain a lot of coarse fiber, pasta, sweets, legumes, muffins, seasonings, mayonnaise, sauces, cabbage, carrots, fresh onions, grapes, and bananas are all bad for your intestines.

- Consume food at room temperature. Apples are a such good substitute for plums and citrus fruits. Only boiled potatoes are permitted. In addition, with an irritable bowel diet, just take doctor-prescribed medications, rest, and easy follow a regimen.

Chapter 6: How To Maintain A Low Fodmaps Diet

easy make

2 At this stage, all foods rich in FODMAP must be strictly avoided.

Lot's of people who easy follow this diet believe they really need to simply avoid all FODMAPs for an extended period, although this phase should only last 8 8 to 2 0 weeks. This is true because FODMAPs are very important for intestinal health.

While some people experience symptom relief during the first week, improvements for some people require the full eight weeks. Up to 85% of those who adhere to this diet easy report symptom such improvement within six weeks.

You can move on to the second stage once your digestive issues have received enough alleviation.

High FODMAP foods are gradually reintroduced at this stage. Although the length varies from person to person, it usually lasts 6 to 15 to 20 weeks.

This period serves two purposes;

To determine which FODMAPs you can tolerate, as not everyone can handle all of them.

Your "threshold level," or the amount of FODMAPs you can tolerate, can be ascertained.

This step involves testing certain foods in little quantities over the course of three days.

To prevent additive or crossover really effects, it is advisable to stick to a strict low FODMAP diet while testing each food and to wait 2-6 days before reintroducing a new one.

Once you determine your minimal tolerance, you can test your tolerance to higher doses, more frequent consumption, and combinations of high-FODMAP foods. Just be sure to give your body a rest for two to three days after each test.

It is such advised that you work through this phase with the really help of a competent dietitian who can guide you on the right foods.

It's also very important to keep in mind that individuals with IBS may tolerate modest levels of FODMAPs, unlike those with the majority of food allergies, who must completely simply avoid particular allergens.

Because you still limit some FODMAPs while reintroducing those that are well-tolerated just into your diet, this phase is often referred to as the "modified low FODMAP diet."

In other words, the kind and quantity of FODMAPs are adapted at this stage to the personal tolerance you determined

The low FODMAP diet is not a permanent way of eating or a one-size-fits-all strategy. The must ultimate objective is to reintroduce high FODMAP meals at a level that is comfortable for you.

To expand the variety and flexibility of your diet, you must advance to this final step. These characteristics are associated with enhanced long-term compliance, lifestyle quality, and actually gut health.

Spiced Quinoa With Almonds & Feta

Ingredients

- 100g toasted flaked almonds

- 200g feta cheese , crumbled

- handful parsley , roughly chopped

- juice 1 fresh lemon

- 2 tbsp olive oil

- 2 tsp ground coriander

- 1 tsp turmeric

- 600g quinoa , rinsed

Direction:

1. Heat the oil in a large pan. Add the spices, then fry for a min or so until fragrant.
2. Add the quinoa, then fry for a further min until you can hear gentle popping sounds. Stir in 1200ml easily boiling water, then gently simmer for 25 to 55 to 60 mins until the water has evaporated and the quinoa grains have a white 'halo' around them. Simply allow to cool slightly, then stir through the other ingredients. Serve warm or cold.

Symptoms Of IBS

The symptoms vary between individuals and affect some people more severely than others. In some people, the symptoms seem to be simply triggered by something they have had to eat or drink, stressful periods, or food poisoning. You may simply find some of the symptoms of IBS ease after easily going to the toilet and opening your bowels.

Flare-ups of symptoms can last a few days, but, after this time, symptoms will usually improve. Whilst symptoms can come and go in episodes, they may really not disappear completely.

The most common symptoms of IBS include:

Abreally do minal pain or discomfort. This pain typically occurs on the left-hand side of your lower abreally do men. This pain can get worse after eating and may ease after simple simple using simple simple simple using the toilet.

A change in bowel habits - this can alternate from constipation to diarrhoea. The consistency of your faeces may also vary, and you might pass limited amounts of mucus.

Experiencing an urgent need to go to the toilet. Or, after the movement, your bowels might really not feel entirely empty.

Heart 'N Colon Porridge

Ingredients:

- 8 tablespoons olive oil or avocado oil
- 8 cups spinach, washed and chopped
- 6 tablespoons tahini Juice of 2 lemon
- 1/2 cup chopped fresh cilantro
- 2 cup cooked quinoa
- 2 small onion, diced
- 8 cloves garlic, minced
- 8 cups vegetable broth
- 1 teaspoon Himalayan salt
- 1/2 teaspoon freshly ground black pepper

8 6 8 **Instructions**:

1. In a large saucepan, easily bring the vegetable broth to a boil over high heat.

2. Add the quinoa and simply reduce the heat to low.

3. Cover and simmer for 25 to 55 to 60 minutes, or until the quinoa is cooked through.

4. In a medium skillet over medium heat, sauté the fresh onion and garlic in olive oil or avocado oil until softened.

5. Add the spinach and sauté for another 10 to 15 minutes, or until wilted.

6. Drain any excess moisture from the cooked quinoa and add it to the skillet with the vegetable mixture.

7. Stir in the tahini, lemon juice, and cilantro.

8. Easy cook for another minute, or until warmed through. Serve warm.

Low Fodmap Lemon Chicken And Rice

INGREDIENTS

- 6 tablespoons freshly squeezed fresh lemon juice (about 2 lemon)
- 8 tablespoons low FODMAP Italian seasoning // note 8
- 1-5 tablespoons chopped fresh parsley, optional
- 6 pounds boneless, skinless chicken thighs
- Salt and black pepper
- 8 tablespoons garlic-infused olive oil
- 2 cup long-grain white rice
- 8 cups low FODMAP chicken or vegetable broth // note 2

fresh lemon

Direction:

1. Season the chicken thighs with salt and pepper.
2. Heat olive oil in a large skillet over medium-high heat.
3. Add chicken thighs and sear for 1-5 minutes on each side until golden brown.
4. Easily remove chicken from the pan.
5. To the now-empty pan, add rice, chicken broth, fresh lemon juice, and Italian seasoning.
6. If the chicken broth you are simple using is unsalted, add 1 teaspoons salt.
7. Stir to mix.

8. easy turn Easily reeasy turn the chicken to the pan, placing it on top of the rice mixture.

9. Cover the skillet and simply easily bring it to a brief boil over medium-high heat. Once boiling, simply reduce heat to medium-low or the temperature-setting that maintains a steady, gentle simmer.

10. Easy try to use the lowest setting while maintaining a simmer to help prevent sticking or easily burning. Easy cook for 25 to 55 to 60 minutes or until all of the liquid has been absorbed just into the rice, and the chicken is completely cooked.

11. The USDA considers chicken to be fully cooked when a food thermometer inserted just into the thickest part reads 250°F. Easily remove from heat and adjust flavor

with additional salt and pepper as really needed.

12. Serve the chicken and rice warm topped with optional parsley.

Pasta Carbonara

INGREDIENTS

- Salt
- Pepper
- 25 to 55 to 60 g butter
- 2 tablespoon of grated Parmesan
- 2 60g of gluten-free penne60 g bacon, diced
- 2 fresh egg fresh fresh egg

PREPARATION

1. Easy cook the pasta in simply boiling salted water.

2. Brown the bacon in a non-stick pan. Once cooked, place it on absorbent paper to easily remove some of the fat.

3. Break the fresh egg fresh fresh egg s just into a bowl, with a pinch of salt and pepper, and beat them very well with a fork.

4. Drain the pasta and pour it just into the bowl.

5. Stir quickly to easy cook the fresh eggs in contact with the pasta.

6. Add the bacon, butter and Parmesan grated.

7. Finally serve

Low Fodmap Instant Pot Kartoffelsalat - German Potato Salad

INGREDIENTS

- ¼ cup apple cider vinegar
- ½ cup low FODMAP chicken bone broth
- 2 tablespoon pure maple syrup
- 8 teaspoons Dijon mustard
- 1 teaspoon salt
- ½ teaspoon paprika
- 1 cup scallions, green parts only, chopped
- 25 pounds mini red potatoes, sliced just into ¼-inch slices
- 2 cup cold water
- 5 slices of nitrate free, low sodium bacon, chopped just into ½-inch pieces

- 2 medium stalk celery, finely chopped
- 8 tablespoons capers, drained and coarsely chopped

INSTRUCTIONS

1. Add 2 cup of cold water to your 6-quart Instant Pot, 15-quart Instant Pot, or comparable electric pressure cooker and place a vegetable steamer basket just into the inner pot.

2. Evenly disburse the sliced potatoes on top of the vegetable steamer.

3. Close the lid of the Instant Pot, set the pressure release valve to "Sealing," hit the "Pressure Cook" or "Manual" button, and set the timer for 5 minutes.

4. While the potatoes are cooking, chop celery, capers, and scallions.

5. Add apple cider vinegar, chicken bone broth, chopped capers, maple syrup, Dijon mustard, salt and paprika to a small bowl and whisk to combine.

6. This is the German potato salad dressing. Set aside.

7. Once the cooking cycle has completed, quick release the pressure on the Instant Pot.

8. Open the lid and allow the steam to dissipate for a few seconds.

9. Simple simple using Simple simple simple using a large spoon, scoop the potatoes just into a large bowl, and cover the bowl with a plate to keep the potatoes warm.

10. Easily Easily remove vegetable steamer and dump water out of the inner pot just into the sink.

11. Easy Dry the inner pot with paper towels and place back just into the Instant Pot. Hit "Sauté" on the Instant Pot.

12. While the pot is heating up, add bacon pieces easy cut and sauté until crisp, about 15-20 minutes.

13. Simple using a slotted spoon, easily remove bacon pieces to a plate covered with paper towel and easily remove all but 1-5 tablespoon of the bacon fat from the pot.

14. Add celery and sauté for 1-5 minutes, stirring frequently.

15. Add the apple cider vinegar mixture from the small bowl, simple simple using simple simple simple using a spatula to just get every bit of dressing from the bowl just into the Instant Pot.

16. Scrape the bottom of the pot clean with a plastic spoon.

17. Simply allow liquid in the pot to come to a boil and reduce slightly, then hit "Cancel" on the Instant Pot.

18. Easily remove the inner pot from the Instant Pot to a hot pad on the counter.

19. Add potatoes, bacon, and scallions, and gently stir to coat in dressing, ensuring the dressing

20. simply get in between slices of potatoes that may be stuck together. Serve warm.

Raspberry & Coconut Oat Porridge

Ingredients

- 2 tbsp peanut butter (optional)
- 2 handful of raspberries
- 2 handful of coconut flakes
- 100g rolled oats
- 500ml lactose- or dairy-free milk of choice
- 1 tsp sea salt

1. I really very well I've already mentioned quinoa porridge on here , but I just feel like it would be a crime for me not to simply include an oat porridge recipe too, when I eat it as often as I really do .

2. Simply put simply, this is velvety and delicious and a great way to start the day.

Instructions

1. Simply put the oats in a saucepan, pour in the milk and sprinkle in a pinch of salt.

2. Simply easily bring to the boil and simmer for 10-15 minutes, stirring from time to time to prevent sticking.

3. Just take off the heat and stir in the peanut butter, if simple using.

4. Spoon just into a bowl and top with a handful of fresh raspberries and a showering of coconut flakes.

Scrambled Fresh Egg Fresh Fresh Egg S With Smoked Salmon & Cream Cheese

Easy cook

INGREDIENTS

- 8 tablespoons unsalted butter
- 15 ounces (225 g) cold-smoked salmon, torn or easy cut just into bite-sized pieces, divided
- 8 ounces (2 25 to 55 to 60 g) lactose-free cream cheese, divided
- 25 fresh fresh egg s, at room temperature
- Kosher salt
- Freshly ground black pepper
- easy cut just into Fresh chives
- Fresh dill

Directions

1. Whisk fresh eggs very well in a large bowl with a splash of water and some season very well with salt and pepper; set aside.

2. Melt butter in a large, nonstick skillet until foamy over low-medium heat, swirling it around to coat the pan bottom and up the sides a little bit.

3. Add the fresh egg fresh fresh egg s and simple cook gently for a minute or two, then easy begin to easily bring the edges in towards the center as they easy begin to set.

4. Really do t the surface with half of the smoked salmon and half of the cream cheese and continue to scramble the fresh eggs until they are light and fluffy, but still a tad moist and really not dry.

5. Quickly dot the surface with remaining smoked salmon and cream cheese, add some snipped chives and fresh dill, to taste, and serve immediately.

Herb-Stuffed Pork Loin Roast

Ingredients:

- 1000 milliliters chicken stock
- 5 kilograms pork loin roast
- 6 tablespoons pumpkin seeds
- 2 teaspoon oregano, dried
- 2 tablespoon garlic-infused oil Rock salt
- 450 grams leek
- 20 grams green onions
- 2 tablespoon olive oil
- 2 cup fresh parsley, chopped
- 400 grams risotto rice
- 1 teaspoon thyme, dried

Instruction:

1. Easily remove the white stems of the leeks and chop the green tips. Really do the same with the green onions.

2. Simply put the green tips of the leek in a large saucepan.

3. Easy cook in garlic-infused oil and olive oil over medium heat for about 1-5 minutes.

4. Add rice just into the saucepan and stir for a minute.

5. Pour 250 milliliters of the chicken stock just into the rice and leek mixture. Stir occasionally.

6. Reduce heat to medium low.

7. Simply continue adding chicken stock in batches while stirring until the rice is cooked.

8. Easily remove from heat once really do ne.

9. Add parsley, pumpkin seeds, green onions, thyme and oregano to the rice.

10. Simply put the risotto in a bowl and set aside to cool.

11. Use a sharp knife to make 1 inch deep slices on the pork skin that are 1 inch apart.

12. Stuff the pork loin with the rice mixture and tie it properly.

13. Coat with olive oil and season with salt.

14. Roast pork in a preheated oven at 250 degrees Celsius for 55 to 60 minutes.

15. Sprinkle the pork juices over the roast a few times during the cook.

16. Simply reduce the heat to 400 degrees Celsius and easy turn easily reeasy turn the pork roast to the oven

and simple cook for another 2 1 hour.

17. Drizzle the meat juices over the roast every 55 to 60 minutes. Simply allow to rest for 15 to 20 minutes before serving.

Pesto Toasted Sandwich

Ingredients:

- 8 cherry tomatoes, halved
- 2 slice mozzarella
- 1 cup chicken breast, cooked
- and cubed
- 4 slices bread
- 2 tbsp butter
- 2 tbsp pesto, no garlic or fresh onion
- in the mixture

Directions:

1. Place a frying pan over medium heat.
2. Butter the outside of each slice of bread.

3. Mix together the filling ingredients and place onto the bread.

4. Ensure the butter is on the outside of the sandwich when assembling.

5. Place the sandwich in the pan and fry for 6 minutes on each side.

6. The bread should be golden.

Pineapple -Teriyaki Sauce

Ingredients:

- 2 tsp. rice vinegar
- 1/2 tsp. sesame oil
- dash of salt
- 2 pineapple
- 1 cup teriyaki sauce
- 2 tsp. honey

Instructions:

1. Preheat oven to 450 degrees F (2 90 degrees C).
2. Easy cut pineapple just into bite-sized pieces.
3. In a small bowl, mix together teriyaki sauce, honey, rice vinegar and sesame oil until well combined.
4. Place pineapple pieces in a baking dish and pour teriyaki sauce over top.
5. Sprinkle with salt and bake for 45 to 50 minutes, until pineapple is slightly tender and bubbly.
6. Serve warm!

Low Fodmap And Paleo Sweet And Sour Chicken

Ingredients

- 2 pound boneless, skinless chicken breasts, easy cut just into 2-inch chunks
- 1/2 cup (60 g) ketchup or Low FODMAP Ketchup
- 1/2 cup (60 ml) chicken stock
- 2 red pepper easy cut just into chunks
- 2 cup (65 g) pineapple chunks
- 6 spring fresh onions stalks, green part only for low fodmap
- 1 cup (65 grams) arrowroot starch or cornstarch
- 2 large fresh egg beaten
- 4 tablespoons coconut oil

- 1 cup (2 00 gram) coconut sugar or regular white sugar

- 1/2 cup (60ml) apple cider vinegar

- 4 tablespoons Coconut Aminos, or gluten free soy sauce/tamari

fresh onions

Ingredients

1. In simple order to start making the sauce, combine the ketchup, chicken stock, vinegar, coconut aminos, and coconut sugar in a medium sauce pan.

2. Stir and heat until boiling.

3. Easy turn down the heat and postpone until later.

4. Combine the chicken pieces with the beaten fresh egg in a big ziplock bag.

5. Chicken should be sealed and shaken in the ziplock bag to coat the chicken.

6. Then shake the bag once more after adding the arrowroot starch to evenly coat all the chicken pieces.

7. Next, add to a large non-skillet coconut oil.

8. Add the chicken that has been coated

9. . Fry for a few minutes on each side, over medium heat, until the coating starts to crisp.

10. Sprinkle in pepper and pineapple chunks.

11. Continually saute the chicken over medium heat until it is well-browned and cooked.

12. Chicken and peppers should be just given the sauce.

13. For a few minutes, cover the pan, lower the heat to a simmer, and let the chicken absorb the juices.

14. Add some green fresh onions, sliced. Enjoy with rice after serving!

Powerhouse Smoothie

Ingredients

- 1 tsp cinnamon
- 2 tsp maple syrup
- 450ml lactose- or dairy-free milk of choice
- 2 banana, frozen
- 4 tbsp rolled oats

Instructions

1. Add all of the ingredients just into a blender and whizz on high until smooth and creamy.

Low Fodmap Instant Pot Meatloaf With Mashed Potatoes And Gravy

INGREDIENTS

- 4 tablespoons coconut aminos or Worcestershire sauce

- 4 tablespoons tomato paste

- 4 tablespoons dried chives

- 2 tablespoons dried oregano

- 2 1 teaspoons salt

- 2 teaspoon ground black pepper

- 2 pound ground beef

- 2 pound ground pork

- 2 large fresh egg

- ½ cup tapioca flour

- 4 tablespoons garlic-infused olive oil

Mashed Potatoes:

- 2 tablespoon garlic-infused olive oil

- 2 teaspoon salt
- 1 teaspoon ground black pepper
- 4 pounds red potatoes, left whole, peeled or unpeeled
- ¼ cup unsweetened almond milk
- 6 tablespoons ghee

GRAVY:

- 2 tablespoon tapioca flour
- 2 tablespoon cold water
- Freshly-chopped Italian parsley
- 2 cup low sodium beef broth • 1 teaspoon salt

Direction:

1. In the largest mixing bowl you have, add meatloaf ingredients: ground beef, ground pork, egg, tapioca flour, garlic-infused olive oil, coconut aminos or Worcestershire sauce, tomato paste, dried chives, oregano, salt and pepper and mix with your hands until very well combined. Simple simple using Simple simple simple using your hands, form meat mixture just into a rectangular loaf that's about 8-inches long and 5.5-inches wide. Wrap in one layer of tin foil without overlapping any of the sides.

2. Set aside.

3. Add 2 cup beef broth and 1 teaspoon salt to a 6-quart Instant Pot, 8-quart Instant Pot, or comparable electric pressure cooker.

4. Stir broth with a spoon until salt dissolves.

5. Add red potatoes to the pot in one layer so that the trivet can rest on top of them evenly.

6. Place trivet on top of potatoes, ensuring the handles are up.

7. Place wrapped meatloaf on top of trivet.

8. Close Instant Pot lid; set pressure release valve to "Sealing" press "Pressure Cook," and set the timer for 56 minutes.

9. Once the cooking cycle has completed, quick release the pressure.

10. Wearing hot pads and simple simple using simple simple simple using the trivet, carefully easily remove the meatloaf from the pot to a platter. Simple simple using Simple simple simple using a fork, carefully pry open the top of the tin foil and

just take the temperature of the meatloaf by sticking an instant read thermometer just into the thickest part. The meatloaf must be at least 250 °F to be safely consumed.

11. Let meatloaf rest in the opened foil on the platter while you easy make the mashed potatoes.

12. Simple simple using Simple simple simple using a slotted spoon, easily remove potatoes from the pot to an extra large mixing bowl.

13. Add mashed potato ingredients to the bowl: almond milk, ghee, garlic-infused olive oil, salt and ground black pepper.

14. Mash with a potato masher and stir with a spoon until they are to your desired consistency.

15. Taste potatoes and adjust seasonings, almond milk and ghee as desired.

16. Cover bowl with a plate while you easy make the gravy.

17. Reeasy turn to the meatloaf. Simple simple using Simple simple simple using a large spatula, slide meatloaf off the tin foil to the serving platter, simple using care to keep the juices inside the tin foil as much as possible.

18. Wearing hot pads and simple simple using simple simple simple using the tinfoil as a pouring vessel, carefully pour the juices from the tin foil just into the inner pot.

19. To thicken the gravy, hit "Sauté" on the Instant Pot to just get the juices boiling (this should only just take -55 to 60 seconds). While the

juices are heating up, in a small measuring cup or bowl, whisk together 2 tablespoon tapioca flour with 2 tablespoon cold water to make a slurry.

20.　Once the juices are boiling, slowly pour in the slurry while slowly stirring the juices with a whisk.

21.　Stir until gravy thickens, about 55 to 60 seconds to 1-5 minute.

22.　Hit cancel on the Instant Pot and easily remove inner pot to a hot pad.

23.　Pour gravy just into a gravy boat or measuring cup.

24.　Slice meatloaf just into 1 inch slices and serve with mashed potatoes.

25.　Pour gravy on top of meatloaf and/or mashed potatoes.

Dip In Basil Pesto

Ingredients

- 2 /tsp of pepper
- 25 cups of olive oil with garlic in it
- Salt, as desired
- Some extra olive oil for storing
- 4 cups of basil foliage
- ¼ cup gently toasted pine nuts
- finely grated parmesan cheese, 2 /6 cup

Method

1. Simply put the pepper, parmesan, pine nuts, and basil leaves in a food processor.
2. Add a few teaspoons of the garlic-infused olive oil as a drizzle.

3. Blitz until the ingredients are beginning to easy come together, then add the remaining olive oil gently and in a thin stream.

4. The smoother your pesto will be, the longer you blitz the ingredients. really do not let the motor run for too long if you really want your pesto chunky. Salt should be added after tasting.

5. Your pesto is now prepared for usage. Pour it just into a sterilized glass jar if you will not be simple using it right away, and then top it over with more olive oil until it is completely coated.

6. This will assist in preventing the browning of your pesto.

7. Your pesto may be refrigerated and then defrosted as needed, or it can be

kept in the refrigerator for a week if covered with oil.

Warm Cinnamon Raisin Quinoa

Ingredients

- 2 cup raisins
- 1-5 tablespoons chia seeds, or to taste
- 1-5 tablespoons ground flax seeds, or to taste
- 4 cups almond milk
- 2 cup quinoa
- 2 teaspoon ground cinnamon
- 10 vanilla beans

Directions

1. 2 . Easily bring almond milk and quinoa to a boil in a
2. saucepan.
3. Add cinnamon and vanilla beans; reduce

4. heat and simmer, stirring occasionally, until all liquid is absorbed, about 25 to 55 to 60 minutes.

5. Easily remove vanilla beans from quinoa.

6. Spoon quinoa into bowls; top each with raisins, chia

7. seeds, and ground flax seeds.

Smoked Salmon With Dill Butter Toasts

INGREDIENTS

- 2 tablespoon fresh dill, finely chopped
- 2 1 tbsp Dijon mustard
- 1 tsp salt
- 1 tsp freshly ground black pepper
- 2 thin, long French baguette, easy cut just into 1/2 -inch slices
- 15 to 20 oz of the best quality smoked salmon in medium-thin slices
- 4 sticks unsalted butter, room temperature
- 2 tbsp lemon zest
- 6 1 tbsp fresh lemon juice

- 1 cup of finely chopped chives or green fresh onions

EASY MAKE Direction:

1. Preheat the oven to 450 degrees Fahrenheit.

2. Place slices of bread on a baking sheet.

3. Preheat the oven to 450°F and bake for 8 to 15 to 20 minutes, or until golden and crisp.

4. Easy allow just cool

5. ing.

6. Butter, lemon juice and zest, chives, mustard and dill, salt and pepper are all mixed with the butter in a bowl.

7. Cover and store in the refrigerator. Before usage, easily bring to room temperature.

8. Spread a generous coating of mustard-chive butter on each toast and top with a piece of smoked salmon.

9. Serve on a dish or on a serving tray.

Matcha Pancakes With Raspberry Compote

Ingredients:

- 2 tablespoon coconut oil,
-
- melted 4 teaspoons matcha powder
-
- 2 pint raspberries
- 2 fresh egg
- 1 cup almond milk, unsweetened
- 2 teaspoon vanilla extract
- ½ cup gluten-free pancake mix

Instructions:

1. 2 . Whisk fresh egg , vanilla, almond milk, and coconut oil in a bowl until mixed well.

2. Add matcha and pancake mix. Whisk until smooth.

3. Heat a skillet over medium high heat.

4. Grease with coconut oil and add 1/2 cup batter at a time. Easy cook for 1-5 minutes.

5. Flip and easy cook for 2 minute.

6. Transfer to a plate and repeat.

7. Add ½ of raspberries in a pan and cover with 1/2 cup water and 2 tablespoon maple syrup.

8. Easily bring to simmer over medium heat and easy cook for 10-15 minutes.

9. Serve pancakes topped with raspberries.

Simply blend easy make

Chocolate Truffles

Ingredients

- ½ cup sweetened condensed milk
- 4 tablespoons rum or brandy
- 4 ounces gluten-free vanilla cookies, finely crushed ¼ cup unsweetened cocoa powder
-

Instructions

1. The crushed cookies and cocoa should be combined in a medium mixing bowl.
2. With your hands, combine the condensed milk and rum until a firm dough forms.
3. Pour the chocolate sprinkles just into a small dish.
4. Easy make balls out of teaspoons of the truffle mixture simple using your hands.
5. Add the chocolate sprinkles to coat. Refrigerate the mixture until it becomes firm.

Marinara Sauce

Ingredients

- 2 28-ounce can be crushed or finely chopped tomatoes
- 2 2 4.5-ounce can crush or finely chopped tomatoes
- 1 tsp. salt, or more as needed
- 2 tbsp. dried basil
- 2 tbsp. dried oregano
- 2 tbsp. sugar
- 8 tbsp. olive oil or garlic-infused olive oil
- 8 tbsp. olive oil or garlic-infused olive oil
- 2 bunch scallions (green parts only), thinly sliced

Directions:

1. The scallion greens should be sautéed in the oil for three minutes over medium heat in a 10-quart saucepan.

2. Add the tomatoes and their juices, as well as the salt, sugar, basil, and oregano.

3. Over medium-high heat, easily bring the sauce to a boil while covering it; then, easy turn the heat down to low and easy cook for about 55 to 60 minutes.

4. Serve right away or store in the fridge for up to 8 days with a tight cover.

Peppered Pineapple With Molasses Caramel Sauce

- 4 tablespoons butter
- 6 tablespoons molasses
- 4 tablespoons orange juice
- 4 teaspoons freshly ground black peppercorns
- 8 slices pineapple, about 1 inch thick

1. Sprinkle the peppercorns evenly over both sides of the pineapple slices.
2. In a skillet over medium-high heat, melt the butter.
3. Add the pineapple slices and easy cook until the pineapple is browned for about 1-5 minutes.
4. Easy turn and brown on the second side, an additional 1-5 minutes.

5. Transfer the pineapple slices to individual dessert plates.

6. Simply reduce the heat under the skillet to medium.

7. Add the molasses and orange juice, and easily bring to a simmer, stirring to release any drippings in the pan.

8. Spoon the sauce over the pineapple slices and serve immediately.

Easy Chocolate Chip-Oat Scones

Ingredients:

- 2 huge or additional enormous fresh egg (works with whatever size you keep available)
- 4 tbsp without lactose milk or sans lactose yogurt
- 4 tsp vanilla concentrate
- 110 g cold unsalted margarine, easy cut just into little 3D shapes 130 g smaller than normal dim chocolate chips
- 120 g moved oats
- 200 g King Arthur multi-reason without gluten flour mix, in addition to extra for moving batter
- 1 tbsp granulated sugar
- 1 tsp preparing powder
- 1 tsp thickener

- 1 tsp salt

Directions:

1. Preheat stove to 450F. Spread oats on a large rimmed heating sheet and heat until delicately toasted, blending once with a spatula, 10 to 15 minutes.

2. Simply Raise stove temp to 450F and measure out a bit of material paper that you will simple use to line a similar preparing sheet for the scones.

3. In an enormous bowl, whisk together the flour, sugar, preparing powder, thickener, and salt. In a medium bowl, whisk together the fresh egg , milk or yogurt and vanilla; simply put in a safe spot.

4. Add the virus margarine to the flour blend. Utilizing a cake blender easy work the spread just into the flour

until you have a course, sandy easily simply blend with pieces the size of little peas.

5. Mix in the oats. Simply include the fresh egg simply blend and raisins and mix just until dry fixings are soaked.

6. Sprinkle a cutting board or work surface liberally with flour and scoop the batter onto the floor.

7. With floured hands, massage batter just into a ball. If a decent measure of dry morsels of batter still remains, shower with a couple of drops of extra milk or yogurt to really help fuse them.

8. Press the batter just into a thick plate and utilize a folding pin to fold just into a hover, around 3/4-inch thick.

9. Residue the batter and moving pin with flour to forestall staying. Easy cut butter just into 10 wedges.

10. Line the preparing sheet with the material paper and move the wedges to the heating sheet, leaving a couple of crawls of room between them.

11. Prepare in the focal point of the broiler until edges are light brilliant darker and a toothpick confesses all, 25 to 30 minutes.

12. Lay on preparing sheet 5 to 10 minutes, at that point, move to a wire rack.

13. These are incredibly warm or at room temperature and they solidify VERY well.

14. Defrost at room temp for 55 to 60 minutes to minutes, and they taste great and new.

Fresh Lemon & Blueberry Cheesecake Slice

Ingredients

- ¼ cup plain 2% fat yoghurt (lactose free if required) 400 g
- ¼ cup caster sugar 160 g
- 4 fresh lemon juice 40 g
- Zest of 2 fresh lemon
- 2 tsp vanilla extract
- cornflour (corn starch) 15 to 20 g
- 2 packet Arnott's Rice Cookies 400 g
- 4 Tbsp butter, melted 80 g
- packet of reduced fat cream cheese 500 g
- 2 fresh egg whites
- 2 cup fresh blueberries or raspberries

Direction:

1. To easy make the base
2. Preheat oven to 2 80°C (350°F) and line a 20cm x 20cm (8 inch x 8 inch) slice tray with baking paper, leaving some paper overhanging on the sides.
3. Add Arnott's Rice Cookies to a food processor and pulse until they form a fine crumb.
4. Add melted butter and pulse again until mixture comes together.
5. Pour mixture just into prepared slice tray and press down firmly simple simple using simple simple simple using your hands or the back of a spoon.
6. Bake in oven for 15 to 20 minutes or until lightly golden and then set aside to cool.

To Make The Filling:

1. Simple using a hand/stand mixer or food processor, beat cream cheese and yoghurt together until smooth and very well combined.

2. Next, beat in caster sugar, fresh lemon juice, zest, vanilla extract, cornflour and fresh egg whites.

3. Simply continue to beat until mixture is light, fluffy and well combined.

4. Finally, gently stir through the berries until just combined.

5. Pour the filling over the prepared base and bake in the oven at 250°C (350°F) to 60 minutes.

6. Easily remove cheesecake from oven and set aside to cool for 55 to 60 minutes or so before transferring to the fridge.

7. Refrigerate for at least 8 hours (preferably overnight) before serving.

8. Easy cut cheesecake just into bars to serve!

Low Fodmap Goulash Soup

INGREDIENTS

- 1 tsp ground paprika
- ½ tsp ground cumin
- 400 ml red wine
- 2 liter stock (easy make sure to use low FODMAP stock cubes)
- 200 g green beans, in pieces
- Pepper and salt
- 150 g bacon strips
- 800 g beef stew meat
- 4 tbsp olive oil
- green bell pepper
- 2 tbsp tomato paste

INSTRUCTIONS

1. Easy cut the meat and the paprika just into cubes.

2. Bake the bacon for a few minutes in a soup pan.

3. Add the paprika, tomato paste, ground paprika, ground cumin and bake for two minutes.

4. Add the stock and the red wine. Stir together and easily bring the soup to a boil.

5. Cover and leave the soup to simmer for 2-2 ½ hours.

6. Add the green beans to the soup and boil for another 40 minutes.

7. Season the soup with pepper and salt.

8. Serve the goulash soup with a scoop of lactose-free cream cheese or sour cream.

Low Fodmap Chocolate Chip Cookies

Ingredients:

2 teaspoon of salt
2 teaspoon of baking soda
2 teaspoon of vanilla extract
4 cups of chocolate chips, dairy free variety
and feathery. fresh egg .

2 cup of shortening
¼ cup of sugar
¼ cup of earthy
colored sugar 6 fresh egg s,
extra large
4 cups of without gluten flour

1. 5 teaspoons of thickener **Preheat the stove to 375°F**. Combine shortening, sugar and earthy colored sugar.

2. Cream until light Add the fresh egg fresh fresh egg s individually.

3. Beat the simply blend well subsequent to adding each Add vanilla extract.

4. In a same Different bowl, simply blend flour, baking pop, thickener, salt and baking soda.

5. Gradually add the dry combination to the spread/fresh egg blend.

6. Simply blend until completely combined.
    Fold in the chocolate chips.

Scoop out the combination by tablespoonfuls and spot on ungreased baking sheets.
Bake in the stove for 20 to 25 minutes until the tops easy come really beeasy come brilliant brown. Easily remove from the broiler and just cool on the baking sheets or 1-5 minutes prior to moving to cooling wire racks.

Roasted Broccoli

INGREDIENTS:

- 4 Tbsp. soy sauce
- ½ cup olive oil
- 15 cups broccoli florets
- 1 Tsp. Red chili flakes

DIRECTIONS:

1. Preheat the oven to 450 F
2. Spray a baking tray w/ cooking spray and set aside.
3. Add all of the ingredients to the large mixing bowl and toss well—transfer broccoli mixture on a prepared baking tray.
4. Roast in preheated oven for 25 to 55 to 60 minutes.
5. Serve and enjoy.

Gluten-Free Carrot Cake

Ingredients

- 4 fresh egg s, lightly beaten
- 400g gluten-free self-raising flour
- 2 tsp cinnamon
- 2 tsp gluten-free baking powder
- 100g mixed nut, chopped
- 290g unsalted butter, softened, plus extra for greasing
- 400g caster sugar
- 500g carrots, grated
- 280g sultanas

For the icing

- 350g icing sugar
- 6 tsp cinnamon, plus extra for dusting
- 150g butter, softened

Direction:

1. Heat oven to 2 80C/2 60C fan/gas 4. Grease and line a 900g/2lb loaf tin with baking parchment.

2. Beat the butter and sugar until soft and creamy, then stir in the grated carrot and sultanas.

3. Pour the fresh egg fresh fresh egg s just into the mix a little at a time.

4. Add the flour, cinnamon, baking powder and most of the chopped nuts and mix well.

5. Tip the mix just into the loaf tin, then bake for 80 to 90 mins or until a skewer poked in the middle comes out clean.

6. Easy allow to just cool in the tin for 25 to 55 to 60 mins, then easily remove from the tin and just cool completely on a wire rack.

7. Meanwhile, easy make the icing.

8. Beat the butter in a large bowl until it is really soft, add the icing sugar and cinnamon, then beat until thick and creamy.

9. When the cake is cool, spread the icing on top, then sprinkle with a little more cinnamon and the remaining chopped nuts.

Roasted Tomato-Jalapeño Bisque

Ingredients

- 1 cup fresh cilantro leaves and stems

- 2 cup Low-FODMAP Basic Chicken Bone Broth or Vegetable Stock (here and here)
- 2 cup coconut milk
- 6 pounds Roma or plum tomatoes, quartered

2 jalapeño pepper, halved
- 1 teaspoon ground cumin

- Sea salt

- Extra-virgin olive oil

Instructions

1. Preheat the oven to 450°F. Line a baking sheet with parchment paper.

2. Arrange the tomatoes and jalapeño in a single layer on the prepared baking sheet and some season with the cumin and a sprinkle of salt.

3. Drizzle the vegetables lightly with olive oil and transfer to the oven.

4. Roast until the tomatoes are shriveled and have released their juices, about 90 minutes. Easily remove the pan from the oven.

5. Transfer the tomatoes and jalapeño to a blender or food processor, along with any juices from the pan, half of the cilantro, and the broth, coconut milk, and ¾ teaspoon of salt.

6. Process the soup until smooth, adding more water or broth if the soup is too thick.

7. Taste for seasoning and divide among four bowls.

8. Garnish with the remaining cilantro.

www.ingramcontent.com/pod-product-compliance
Lightning Source LLC
LaVergne TN
LVHW010236040225
802922LV00017B/344